How
I
Quit Smoking
and
Lived
To Tell About It!

Other books by Mel Calvert

Bertha's Battle

*A Funny Thing Happened To Me
On The Way To My Funeral*

How
I
Quit Smoking
and
Lived
To Tell About It!

Revised Edition

The **Quit Smoking Program** Sensation
7 Steps to Life
and the Story Behind It

MEL CALVERT

"We hope that this donation will help you get started, and that your efforts do help kids avoid smoking. My father started when he was nine; he died from throat cancer at the age of 65, three months after walking me down the aisle; his wife died at 57, also of throat cancer.

Thank you for your good work. I'm glad that my work can help in this effort."

DEDICATION

~

To my family, both past and present

~

CONTENTS

FOREWORD

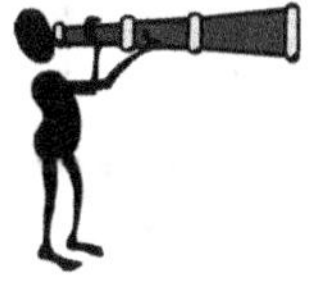

SEVERAL years ago, I was speaking to a convention of school administrators. After my talk, I was approached by two men with the intention, I thought, of congratulating me on my speech. One was tall and young and wore a polo shirt with a distinct emblem on the pocket with the initials SCAT. The other, a far more mature "young" man, was short, well dressed in a business suit and had a rather distinguished air about him. As it turned out, the congratulations did come, but not in the manner to which I had long been accustomed.

The mature gentleman looked me directly in the eye as he took my hand and said, "Dr. Rohm, you are just the person we need to help us to keep kids from starting to smoke." The two of them ganged up on me, took me to a seat in the lobby and proceeded to show me their wonderful program called Student Crusade Against Tobacco. This was my first meeting with Mel Calvert and his young son, Michael. We spent a delightful hour together during which I agreed to join their Board of Advisors. I was impressed not only with their sincerity and commitment, but also with their wit and humor.

Today, even as I write this, I am winging my way to Poland to address a group of business people and have just finished reading the manuscript for this book. If you enjoy laughing, then you will enjoy this excellent new work. Mel has an unusual way of getting us to laugh at ourselves while we learn new information. Anyone who has secretly wished they could kick the nicotine habit but has not been able to do so will love this book.

Someone once said, "When the student is ready, the teacher will appear." Well, the teacher has arrived!

— Dr. Robert Rohm

Dr. Robert Rohm, Ph.D., is founder and president of Personality Insights, Inc., Atlanta, Georgia. He is a renowned author, educator, popular corporate trainer and keynote speaker. He has authored or co-authored many books, including "Positive Personality Profiles" and "Who Do You Think You Are . . . Anyway? " DISCover more at www.personality-insights.com/

PREFACE

Each of these 7 steps has been designed to make quitting as easy as possible. Each is a very important part of the whole. The *7 Steps to Life* program saves you all the research. It is compiled from numerous medical journals, research and personal experience. It puts the most effective steps right at your fingertips!

This book was originally published in 2001, and all proceeds were given to the "Student Crusade against Tobacco," a non-profit organization in Florida, formed to persuade school kids never to smoke. It was paired with the effective media program, "KIK — Kids Influencing Kids."

This second edition has been brought up-to-date with the latest statistics from the same reliable sources as previous and with more testimonials.

If you are a smoker and want to quit, I can promise you that, if you follow *every* step to the letter, you *will* quit —
without climbing the walls!
Please follow the system — it will tell you how to become a **Q**uitter (in the good sense) so that you, too, can . . .

LIVE TO TELL ABOUT IT!

Yours truly,

Mel Calvert

P.S. Here is one reason why the battle is still raging —

"In 1900, one in five Americans died from tuberculosis; TB control succeeded dramatically in reducing this disease. Today, one in five Americans dies from tobacco, but a tobacco industry's marketing budget of billions of dollars per year encourages tobacco use."
— Dr. C. Everett Koop, Former U.S. Surgeon General
National Center for Injury Prevention and Control

ACKNOWLEDGMENTS

"How do I love thee, let me count the ways . . ."

THIS opening line to Elizabeth Barrett Browning's beautiful sonnet best expresses my dilemma in acknowledging the hundreds of people who have positively influenced my life.

Some, of course, are easy. My mother and father, my brothers, my grandparents - long since removed to a better place, my aunts and uncles on both sides of my family, as well as the cousins by the dozens. Actually, the rest are easy, as well. It's just that it would take an entire book to tell something about each of them.

(But, if this book sells well . . .)

To my children with my first wife — Mara, Todd, Laurie, Rick and Lisa — I hereby set down for the entire world to see my tremendous pride, admiration and unconditional love. No father could be happier or more fulfilled for their accomplishments, which includes the wonderful gang of 17 grandchildren and 20 great-grandchildren they have given me.

While I will accept some of the credit for them, a whole lot must go to their mother, Marge, who is still one of the classiest gals I've known, though we parted so many years ago.

To Dr. Robert Rohm for his splendid FOREWORD; and then to people like Greg and Diane Hemsoth, the Rev. Dan Cody and Rabbi Dov Kintoff who gave their total support to our cause; to Kaye Johnson and Brian Smith, who gave so generously of their time for our children's program; to Bill and Fritzie Kuhlmann who have given me a lifetime of pleasant memories; to Dexter Yeager whom I suspect to be the author of some of the "A. Nonymous" quotes in this book; to Dave Jackson (RIP), my show-biz agent, who told anyone who would listen that I was taking 90% of his salary; to Bob and Sue Candler, who have been with us through all kinds of challenges; to Rev. Denis O'Shaughnessy, whom I believe is a saint; to Professor John Bollinger and his beautiful wife, Margaret, for their counsel and support in trying times; to Ken and Lauri McEachern, for their unwavering friendship and their voices in our church choir; to Wray Edwards (RIP), for his out-of-this-world intellect — all of whom have provided me with such positive examples of selfless dedication to others.

And, of course, to my wife of 46+ years, Sunny, not only for her patience and devotion, but also for her expertise in design and layout which makes the overall look of this program so unique; to her mother Lucille — "*You Picked a Fine Time to Leave Me, Lucille*" — for her spiritual love and guidance; and to all the rest of her family for their ready acceptance of me. And especially to our young son, Michael, who has kept *me* feeling young far beyond expectations.

To all these wonderful people, there are no words to express my indebtedness, gratitude and love.

And so, I acknowledge each and every one of you, as well as those I will regret forgetting to mention. You have made me what and who I am today . . . Deal with it!

INTRODUCTION

NO, not really. If you're reading this it can only mean one of two things: you either want to quit smoking, or you're awfully hard up for something to do. Since you're one of those who actually read forewords in the first place, here are a few thoughts to get you into the right frame of mind.

Mark Twain, the great American humorist, once said, "Quitting smoking is easy. I've done it a thousand times." What possible reason could anyone have had in Twain's era for giving up tobacco since it was so acceptable socially, with little, if any, of the stigma it suffers today? It's only within the last few decades that irrefutable proof has come to light about the terrible risks involved. But even with all that, the insidious nature of the nicotine habit makes it one of the most difficult addictions to kick known to man. You'll learn just why that is in the following pages.

You will not be alone in your effort. I will take you by the hand and — if you do what I teach —

You WILL quit,

You will NOT climb the walls, and

You will NOT even want to stomp on the cat.

I promise.

Now, you can just skip this INTRODUCTION entirely and get to the real meat and potatoes to follow.

Of course, if you've already read it, just skip the part about skipping it entirely.

~

*The fear you let build up in your mind is worse
than the situation that actually exists.*
WHO MOVED MY CHEESE?
Spencer Johnson

~

CHAPTER 1

ADMIT YOU'RE AN ADDICT

"HE'S GOT A MONKEY ON HIS BACK."
1930s term describing a drug addiction.

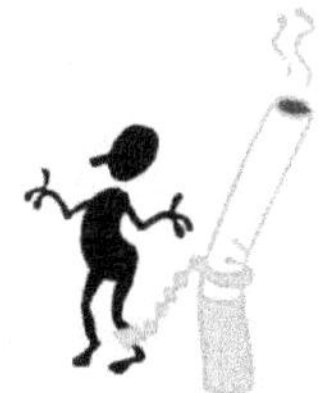

WHEN I first started 'smoking' dried corn silk rolled up in toilet paper or dried horseweeds cut to the right length, it never really occurred to me that my life one day would revolve so consistently around helping other people to quit smoking. Of course, at that age, eight or nine, not much of anything really occurred to me on my own.

Like any country kid, my world was a combination of family, farming, fighting with my two younger brothers — (the local grocer, Al Witt, called us Art, Bart and Fargo), feeding the flocks, fishing, fending off females of any age, flipping pennies to see who got the closest to the line in the dirt, floating down the river during flood stage, flicking flies with a rubber band, feasting at festive family reunions at my father's father's house who was one of the first Ford dealers in the state of Ohio. (Whew! That's a lot of *Fs!)*

My grandmother on my father's side was a fine, Christian lady who lived her entire life doing anything she could for others without asking or expecting anything in return. My grandfather was also a strong, spiritual person, Everyone in the family called him "Poppy" — I think I was the one who named him when I was three or four years old. He worked early on for the State of Indiana as a highway superintendent and supervised the first paving of many of the roads in southeastern Indiana. Serving the community as Sunday School superintendent, city councilman and civic leader, he remains a giant of a man in my memory, both in stature and in character.

Some of my sweetest early childhood memories are from that little conclave of two houses in New Trenton, Indiana, — ours was the tiny cottage down the gravel road, about 200 yards from the big main house of my grandparents. Between the two lay a field of alfalfa which Uncle Bernard would mow every fall, with me riding on the seat beside him. Suddenly, he would shout "Rabbit!" And we would both jump off the tractor to chase down a young bunny whose cover was rapidly falling to the mean old mower.

This same uncle, accompanied by his best buddy, Price Seymour, would wheel me in a little "Taylor Tot" down to the Whitewater River where I got my first taste of fishing. 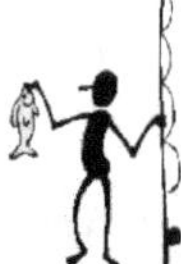

Ah, those **childhood memories** . . .

~ Lying on our backs looking for identifiable cloud formations,

~ Playing, hot and sweaty in the hay mow (strange, we "moe" the hay and put it up in a "maow"),

~ Picking the super-sweet peaches off the small tree by our house, not the little ones, mind you, but those beauties like the ones that come from South Carolina today,

~ Walking barefoot on the gravel road and not even noticing the sharp stones because of the calluses we had developed on the bottoms of our feet,

~ Waving to the train as it sped by our house a few hundred feet down the bank,

~ Playing baseball barefooted in the cow pasture and feeling the warm manure squish between our toes as we ran back to catch a fly ball,

~ Futilely scrubbing hands stained purple from the mulberries, or black from the two huge black walnut trees in front of our house,

~ Running to catch the school bus since we had to walk over a mile to the pickup point — (in the snow and rain, into the wind, uphill both ways!).

It's hard to realize that the uncle I fell in love with when I was five, this "giant" who could do anything — catch wild rabbits with his bare hands, drive a tractor, milk a cow, throw a bale of hay around like it was nothing — was just 17 years old then. I still idolize him and will cherish his memory until I meet up with him again in the great alfalfa field beyond.

~

NEITHER he nor any of my other uncles or aunts, nor my grandparents, nor my parents were smokers. What happened to me? Simple. It was legal. And the social norm. By the time I was ready to graduate from high school where I was a big duck in a little pond athletically, we had moved just across the border to Harrison, Ohio. Because of my involvement in sports, I didn't really get hooked on nicotine until shortly after I graduated from Harrison High School.

This isn't to say that there weren't times when I smoked cigarettes. Bill, my best friend, and I were having a casual cigarette behind the grandstand on the football field when we were somehow spotted by our coach, J.R. Swisher. Now, there's a name for you! Swisher Sweets are very popular today among the younger, "cooler" crowd of juveniles. I doubt if Coach Jesse R. Swisher had any idea he would be immortalized in a cloud of smoke. Of course, I don't have a lot of room to talk. "Calvert" would grab the attention of any wino as long as it was in a bottle.

Anyway, since I was a grade ahead of Bill — (Who-Retired-as-President-of-The-Board-of-Health-in-a-Major-City-Which-Shall-Remain-Nameless-Even-Though-I-attended-the-Conservatory-of-Music-There-and-My-Mother-was-The-Head-Nurse-of-Bethesda-Hospital-up-on-Reading-Road-and-the-Reds-Were-Our-Favorite-Baseball-Team-for-Many-Many-Years), I got the blame for leading him astray and "teaching him how to smoke," which was a big crock, since he was the only person I have ever known in my life who brought along his dad's cigarette roller on camping trips!

But, still, it was me who got the blame for being a bad influence on innocent "Koolie," which was his nickname because it was sort of the way his last name started but, since I don't want to embarrass him, I won't tell it.

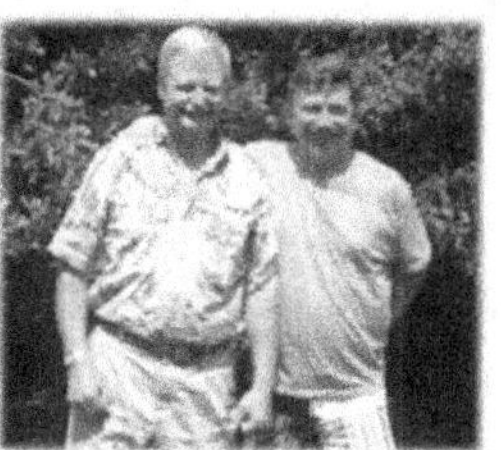

Here's "Koolie" and the author, joined at the hip since childhood.

*Thanks, Bill, for always being there **for** me and being there **with** me, through thick and thin, together or miles apart. My best friend ever!*

~

SPEAKING of names, I doubt if there ever was, or is today, any town in our country with funnier names than what we grew up with:

> ~ Paul Wiwi (pronounced Weewee)
> ~ Shorty Scheich (Shike)
> ~ Mercer Greenham (Grinnum)
> ~ Fuzzy Metler
> ~ Dale Acra (Aikree)
> ~ Pood Offield and Pood Seeley
> ~ Dabber, Tuter and Worm Kober
> ~ John Schott & Ruth Fell (they were an "item")
> ~ Alice Hodap,
>   and the Grand Prize, Winner-Take-All, has to be . . .
> ~ Rosy White.

"Nothing funny about 'Rosy White'," you say? And you're right. However, Rosy set the gossip tongues a-waggin' in our little town of some 1,900 souls when, shortly after graduating from high school (a year or two ahead of me), she up and married the science teacher. Today, he would probably have been prosecuted for contributing to the delinquency of a minor, but, then, it was just too funny for anyone to worry about such a thing, since the science teacher that Rosy White married was a very dapper and learned fellow named Carl Butt and she was known ever after as "Rosy White Butt."

True!

~

IT had never occurred to me to be concerned in the least about being addicted. We already had all the excuses that people still use today:

"I enjoy smoking."
"It relaxes me."
"Everybody else is doing it."

And the thing is, almost everybody *was* doing it. I doubt if there are any reliable statistics available for the number of smokers in the '30s and '40s, but, if my memory is any good at all, I really believe non-smokers were a minority when I was growing up.

I can vividly remember being fascinated by cigarettes, perhaps because my family was very much opposed to putting any form of foreign substance into our bodies, especially alcohol. It was, therefore, a forbidden thing — and, therefore, titillating.

~

ONCE, when my little brothers Robert and Freddie and I were playing over the embankment towards the railroad track we found an empty whiskey bottle, empty except for a few drops when you tilted it. I decided that we should test it to see if it really would put horns and a tail on us. Naturally, the most obvious one to taste it would be Robert. He was only four or five at the time and not yet the Professor Emeritus of Political Science that he is today.

Lacking the people skills and ethics then that he sometimes has today — he's a Democrat — he told on me. Dad picked me up, placed me solidly against the wall where he attempted to push it back by using my delicate body as a hammer and gave me to understand that he was not pleased, and that I should never do that again. He then punctuated the lesson by sending me out to cut a switch with which he then flailed away on my bare legs.

I never did *that* again!!

~

SOME of my earliest memories are picking up butts off the street and lighting them and gagging and coughing and having not a clue that my body was trying to tell me something. We really do have a "genius" body, but our brain doesn't seem capable of paying heed in many cases.

~

BY the way, did you know:

~ That the cigarette butts thrown down after smoking are very toxic?

~ That these toxins get filtered into our environmental water supplies?

~ That filtered butts are worse because they are NOT biodegradable??

Today, there is proof beyond the shadow of a doubt for any intelligent person, that tobacco, specifically the modern manufactured brand-name cigarette, is still the **number one cause of preventable deaths in the United States.**

The following facts are not fun to read. Read them anyway.

TOBACCO FACTS AS OF 2018

• Tobacco use is the leading cause of **preventable** illness and death in the United States. It causes heart disease, cardiovascular diseases, many different cancers and also chronic lung diseases, such as emphysema and bronchitis.

• Cigarette smoking causes an estimated **480,000 deaths** each year, more than AIDs, alcohol, car accidents, illegal drugs, murders and suicides **combined**, by a factor of over two-times! [*See graphs in back of book.*]

• Approximately 41,000 of these deaths are due to exposure to **secondhand smoke.**

• **Worldwide**, the smoking epidemic kills more than seven million people a year.

• **Lung cancer** is the leading cause of cancer deaths among both men and women in the United States. Smoking also causes most cases of **chronic obstructive lung disease.**

• Smoking causes **other types of cancer**, including cancers of the lips, throat, mouth, nasal cavity, esophagus, stomach, pancreas, kidney, bladder, cervix and acute myeloid leukemia.

• People who smoke are up to six times more likely to suffer a **heart attack** than nonsmokers, and the risk increases with the number of cigarettes smoked.

• In 2019, approximately 13.7% of U.S. **adults** were cigarette smokers.

• Nearly 6% of **high school students** smoke cigarettes and/or cigars.

• An estimated 27.5% of high school students use **smokeless** tobacco.

The U.S. Surgeon General Jerome M. Adams officially declared **e-cigarette** use, or vaping, among youth an "epidemic." Even if the **vaping** material does not contain nicotine, the oils used to produce the vapor are irritating to the lungs and make it easier for lung disease to become a problem for life.

These facts are not only disturbing to contemplate in themselves, but also to consider the staggering consequences to us as a nation, namely, the enormous and debilitating drain on our economy — tobacco-related ills **cost** the U.S. approximately $170 billion in health care expenditures and more than $150 billion in lost productivity each year, plus $5.6 billion in lost productivity due to second-hand smoke exposure.

And then there's the very personal, much closer-to-home fact: a pack-a-day habit averages $5.00 each day, $150 every month and $1,800 each year! In a few states, the cost is over $7.00 per pack. If you are in one of these states — New York, Rhode Island, Hawaii and Alaska — do the math! And, in New York City, $17.00 a pack!

So, if you've been smoking for 20 years — just think what you could have done with that money that you watched go up in "smoke." I know, the prices have only fairly recently reached that point of inflation. But guess what? It's going to get worse before it gets better. $20 a pack or even more is on the way. Count on it!

~

STEP # 1

Admit You're an Addict!

"MIRROR, MIRROR, ON THE WALL"

THIS will probably be one of the most important conversations you will ever have in your life. And, with the most important person in your life!

So, just how do we go about quitting this thing?

Well, first comes the **desire** to want to quit. If you don't have the desire, don't even bother! Though you wouldn't have read this far if you didn't have it.

After you've made the **decision** to quit, the first positive step to take is to get in front of a mirror, **look yourself in the eye** and say these words:

> "I am an addict. Something has control over me
> and I do not like it."

Please don't bother to say, "Oh, I already know that." There's something therapeutic about saying it out loud to your mirrored-self and saying it with conviction:

> "I am an addict. Something has control over me,
> and I DO NOT LIKE IT!!"

If you will take this step, you're ready for Step 2, which we will go into in great detail in Chapter Two. See you there!

~

Establish the cause — it creates the energy.
A. Nonymous

~

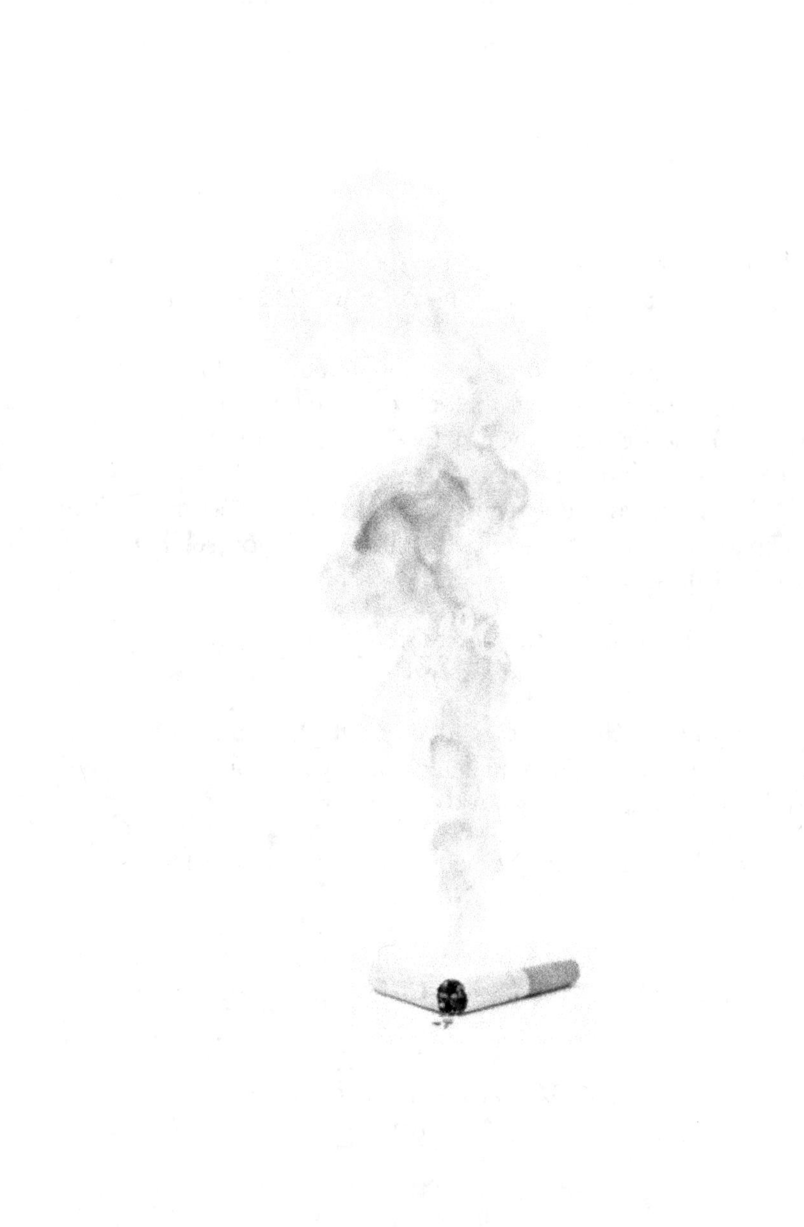

CHAPTER 2

PICK YOUR Q-DAY

WHEN I was just six years old, Poppy, Grandmother, Uncle Bernard and I set off from Harrison in a brand new 1937 Ford four-door sedan. We were on our way to Hollywood where my famous Uncle "Madren" (as he was known in those days) was about to set sail for Hawaii. Come to think of it, he may have already legally changed his name to "John," which wasn't nearly as funny as the rest of the town names. Madren is much funnier.

Anyway, that trip made an indelible impression on me; so much so that I vividly remember scenes much clearer from that trip than some that have occurred within the past few weeks. I hadn't started smoking yet at the age of six, so I didn't have to worry about anyone smelling it on me.

Some of the highlights permanently etched into my memory, but not necessarily in proper order:

~ The wind whistling through the open windows (natural air conditioning)

~ The stop at Grand Canyon. (They say I looked up from the sight after a long pause and asked my Uncle Bernard, "What happened?")

~ The beauty of the Painted Desert

~ The majesty of the Rockies, and

~ The climb in the Ford all the way to the top of Pikes Peak.

I distinctly remember the absence of guard rails on our way up and saw very little of the view from the back floor of the car. I was terrified. And to this day, I suffer from acrophobia — even after earning my jump wings in the 11th Airborne Division and my Private Pilot's license at the same time through a private flying school. I've never been able to overcome my fear of heights, and I still cling, white knuckled, to any support whatever on any height greater than a step ladder. I rejoice that I'm only five feet seven and one-half inches tall!

Our trip consisted of long periods of boring driving, especially through the Midwest. Poppy was appalled to have to stop at a motel and be forced to pay $5.00 for "just a place to sleep." My first impressions upon our arrival in Hollywood were the palm trees and the oil rigs on the outskirts of town. And, my goodness, the awful traffic! We saw more automobiles in California than we had on our entire 2,400-mile trip! Poppy, the Ford dealer, had to have been thinking that he had started his business on the wrong side of the country.

At the pier where we said "Aloha" to Uncle John (aka Madren), I'll always remember the gigantic ocean liner tied to the dock, seemingly with nothing but thousands of paper streamers, and the sound of the beautiful strains of *Aloha-a-e,* and my heart breaking as the ship pulled away leaving me behind. I loved this other uncle, too, and I wanted desperately to go with him.

> *As the sun sails away in the west,*
> *and the ship sinks slowly on the horizon . . .*
> Bugs Bunny

On our way back home, we were flying through the Mojave Desert, windows wide open, when suddenly Uncle Bernard shouted "STOP" and Poppy stomped on the brakes and fought the Ford to a complete stop from the breakneck speed of 50 mph. Uncle Bernard jumped out of the car with his .22 rifle in his hand and ran back a few hundred feet on the highway, warning everyone to "KEEP BACK!" There, draped over a mesquite bush was a real RATTLE SNAKE. He circled it carefully and dispatched it with a total of only 13 shots until it quit moving. The rattles graced Grandmother's what-not shelf for as long as Grandmother and Poppy were alive.

~

SUNDAY dinner was a ritual for the family for many years. Fried Chicken, Mashed Potatoes, Baked Beans, Home-made Bread, Scalloped Corn and, afterwards, good old fashioned, hand-cranked Freezer Ice Cream. Grandmother was always the last one to sit down, having to make trip after trip to and from the kitchen until she was totally satisfied that everything was absolutely perfect.

One such Sunday afternoon, she had made a delivery with a second platter of fried chicken and, not finding an immediate place for it on the table, she put it down on her chair to go back to the kitchen one more time. With everyone moaning, "Please, Mother, let's say the prayer and EAT!" she took one last look around the table while she dried her freshly washed hands on her apron and sat down . . . right on the chicken. Remaining perfectly calm, she picked up the platter and headed for the kitchen to throw it out. But Poppy, ever the problem solver, said, "Mother, you come right back here with that good chicken. There's no need to waste it. You didn't have your dress up, did you?"

~

IT'S been said that **procrastination** is the thief of time. Since someone really did say that, we should all take consolation that putting things off has certainly been done before, and we shouldn't go around acting as though we invented it. However, we should realize that, all things considered —

Procrastination is **not** good.
Doing things *now* — **is** good.

Doing good things, that is. Bad things should be procrastinated the heck out of. Bad things like smoking, for example.

~

STEP # 2

Pick Your Q-Day

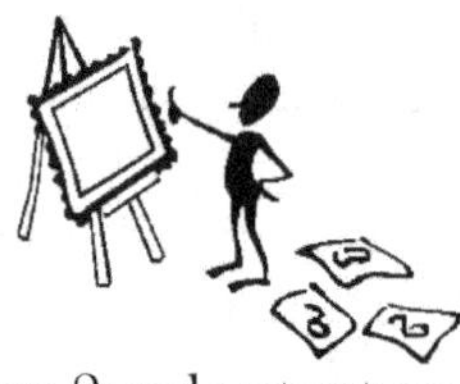

SINCE we're only on Step 2 and not yet ready to actually quit, go ahead and smoke that cigarette you're dying for — (pun intended). Remember that in Step #1, you admitted to yourself that you are an addict. Now, you must make another commitment —

PICK A DAY ON WHICH TO BECOME A *RECOVERING* ADDICT.

We ex-smokers are all addicts for life. Accept it.

Your **Quit Day**, or **Q-Day,** should be a date very easy to remember. A day that you can recall with ease as the day you quit for the rest of your life. Birthdays are great — yours or someone else's. What a wonderful present to give to someone who cares for you. What a wonderful present to give to yourself! Anniversaries are great, too, as well as national holidays, graduation days, or any day which will easily come to mind.

The trick is to pick a day that isn't too close, yet not too far in the future. You don't want your resolve to melt. Two to six weeks would be fine, with three or four being the optimum.

Now, be about it! PICK YOUR Q-DAY and post it all over the house, on mirrors, the fridge, in your car, everywhere! Circle it on your calendar. Write it in your day planner. You're on your way!

~

You don't smoke. The cigarette smokes.
You're just the sucker on the end.
—Zig Zigler

~

Chapter 3

TELL THE WORLD!

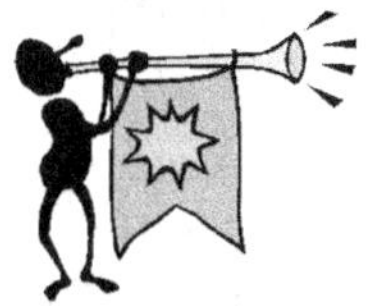

A TEXAN was giving his little boy some fatherly advice.

"Son, never ask a man where he's from. If he's from Texas, you'll know it. If he ain't from Texas, you don't want to embarrass him."

~

A KENTUCKIAN and a Texan were arguing about which of their respective states was the wealthiest.

"Why, in Kentucky, we've got enough gold in Fort Knox to build a 2-ft. high fence all around the whole state of Texas!"

The Texan replied, "You just go ahead and build that fence, sonny, and if I like it, I'll buy it!"

~

A COUPLE of oil-men were walking past a Rolls-Royce dealership in Dallas when one said to the other, "Come on in here with me for a minute. I promised to pick up a car for my wife."

After looking over several with the salesman, the buyer said, "That convertible will be just right. How much do you need?"

"That will be just $225,000 plus tax," he replied.

As the oil-man reached for his check book, his friend whipped out his own check book and said, "Oh, no you don't. You got lunch. This is on me!"

~

TEXAS pride is legendary. With no small amount of justification, I feel. Sam Houston, the Alamo, the Texas Rangers and, yes, even the Dallas Cowboys, conjure up pictures of greatness in the minds of most Americans. A little bit of unraveling of each of these examples, even the jokes, and we find a common thread —

POSITIVE THINKING

Nobody has ever accomplished any lasting success of any kind without a positive attitude. So, how do we get a positive attitude? Are we born with it? Can we learn it? Is there an academic course we can take on the subject?

The answer to each of these questions could actually be "yes."

Some people are born with it. Just think back to when your kids were going through their "terrible twos." They were absolutely, positively certain that they were going to do whatever it was they wanted to do. Period! (Take heart if you are watching your first child go through this stage. The "terrible twos" usually last only until they're twenty-five!)

Can we learn it? Certainly, we can! We *must* learn it if we wish to accomplish anything worthwhile within our lifetime. We need to try to catch ourselves complaining or being negative. My wife, Sunny, has a nickname to match her personality. When people ask her if she ever gets down or depressed, she answers, "Tried it once. Didn't like it."

Are there any academic courses available? I don't know of any actual college courses offered, but there is a plethora of books on the subject. The two most famous and effective, in my opinion, are:

• Dr. Norman Vincent Peal's *The Power of Positive Thinking.*

• Dr. Robert A. Rohm's *Who Do You Think You Are . . . Anyway?*

Read both of these and you can't help but have a positive outlook on everything you do. And, with Dr. Rohm's fascinating concept of personality study, you'll understand yourself and others a lot better, to boot.

~

I REMEMBER, (or at least I think I remember it, since I heard my Grandmother repeat it so often), that I was heading up the road in front of my grandparents' house with a handful of fishing lines and fish hooks. Grandmother looked up from her garden where she was so often absorbed, and asked,

"Whatcha got there?"

I replied, very positively, "Some stickers to catch some fish with."

At the ripe old age of three, I was starting to retrace the three-or four-mile route that Uncle Bernard took when he wheeled me to the Whitewater River. No doubt in *my* mind!

~

ONE of the things that no one ever did, *ever*, in our house, or in my grandparents' house, was go to the bathroom. We didn't have one. Oh, we had a bathtub all right, but relieving one's self was something a civilized person would never do in the house! We had a special place called "the outhouse" to do that kind of stuff. Now, ours was just the ordinary, small one-holer, but my grandparents' outhouse was something to behold. It was a two-holer! One could, and did, make it a social event to "go to the bathroom." My favorite Aunt "TooDoo" and her cousin, Ann Elizabeth, would take me with them while they sat and talked about things young girls talk about. (With their voluminous skirts, nothing ever showed and, at that age, I wouldn't have recognized it if it did.)

It was several years later that the last outhouses disappeared in our part of the country. One of the last to go was Dale Acra's (*A-krees*) in Harrison. The gang often gathered at Knepf's Café — that's pronounced *Neps*, short for Knepfle (pronounced *NEP-lee* - the "f" is silent, like the "p" in swimming . . .). Dale and Mercer Greenham (pr. *Grinnum*) were very much into a few beers, when the argument started over whether or not, on this coming Halloween, anyone could push over Dale's outhouse. The whopping sum of $50 was bet, with a great deal of side money being wagered.

Now, $50 in those days would be the equivalent of around $500 in today's economy. This bet was the subject of much speculation and further argument over the next few weeks. In fact, it was the talk of the town, especially since World War II, Korea, Viet Nam, Desert Storm, the Cincinnati Bengals, and Bernie Madoff were still years away.

Both Dale and Mercer were big men and, looking back, they both kind of remind me of the "Sopranos." Anyway, on Halloween eve of 1940 or '41, Dale sat on his back porch with a big spotlight lighting up his outhouse, a shotgun loaded with rock salt cradled in his lap and a cooler of cold ones by his chair. Mercer had put together a crew of hardy drinkers and young boys just itchin' for adventure and, after giving Dale plenty of time to get into a few brews, came storming down the alley behind Dale's house, which bordered right on the outhouse that Dale had recently walled up with flagstone.

And, despite spotlight, shotgun, rock salt and flagstone, they pushed that sucker over in less time than it took to uncap a Hudepohl. The only casualty of the campaign was Jack Carrroll *(Carol)*. He fell in and did *not* come out smelling like a rose!

~

Your attitude determines your altitude.
Jack Carroll

~

STEP # 3

Tell the World!

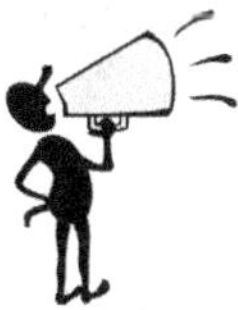

ONE of the best ways there is to have a positive attitude, especially concerning something as frightening as quitting smoking, is to get all the help you can from your friends and loved ones. And the best way to do that is to tell them you're going to quit.

Publish Your Intentions!

Tell the whole world that on [*your Quit-Day*], you are going to quit smoking FOREVER.

First of all, you're going to get the support of the large majority of people, 75%, who don't smoke. Just email your friends, post on your social media accounts, call or write the relatives, talk to the neighbors, co-workers, church friends — talk to everyone! Tell them your Q-Day. You're enlisting the aid of well-wishers, cheer leaders — all your balcony people!

When you talk to them and send out your **Q-Notes**, eMails and posts, you'll find out in a hurry who your true friends are. They will be the ones who say things like:

"Good for you! I know you can do it."
"Great! What can I do to help?"
"I'm here for you! Call me anytime!"

They will be a tremendous support to you in getting over the hump. They'll bolster you up and encourage you through the entire process. Even if they know you've tried to quit before and didn't make it, they'll back you once again.

~

*A true friend is someone who can
make us do what we can.*

*Friends are like walls. Sometimes you lean on them, and
sometimes it's enough just to know they are there.*

Now, you may wish to understand a little better the importance of telling everyone that you're quitting.

• First — there is the natural desire to "save face" by not giving up. With so many people knowing about your **Q-Day**, you'll be more committed to your decision to quit.
• Second — When you add the powerful aid in the support that these positive people will give you, you have a winning combination! By all means, allow them to help!

Remember — The more people you involve, the greater the chances are that you'll quit for good.
It's really surprising how little time it takes for the worst of the **withdrawal symptoms** to go away, and, with the encouragement of a cheering section, it makes it much easier to get through.

~

Now that you have:

   (1) Admitted your Addiction, and
   (2) Picked your Q-Day,
      it's now time to —
   (3) Tell The World!!

COME ON! GO FOR IT!

~

Lift up thy voice like a trumpet!
Is 58

~

20

CHAPTER 4

PICK A Q-BUDDY

As the old saying goes,
> *"You can pick your friends,*
> *and you can pick your nose,*
> *but you can't pick your friend's nose."*

I WONDER if anyone's ever really tried it. I know I haven't ever had that good a friend and I doubt that I ever will. And I know I've never been that good a friend to anyone in my life. Ever!

~

KOOLIE never did get to be *that* good a friend, although we did sit for hours outside my house, sometimes 'til three or four in the morning, in his Dad's blue Plymouth, talking about everything from girls to girls. We both dated a couple of the same ones, at different times, of course, since we weren't nearly as "sophisticated" as the kids are today who can date several in the same night.

We both dated "Bianca" and, as I just said, while we didn't date her at the same time, I'm not sure, looking back in retrospect, that she would have had any problem with it whatsoever. Being a little older than us, "Bianca" was a very adventuresome girl, but we were just too young at 16 to recognize it.

~

ONE of the high spots of my athletic career at Harrison High was the time we beat the future county basketball champs, Green Hills High, 41 to 39, on our home court.

I was a guard, and Koolie, at just about six feet, was as tall as we had. He played center or forward. Our opponents were horribly misshapen fellows who towered over us. Their center was 6-foot-5, and their two forwards were both 6-feet-4 and their guards were both 6-footers.

The way we whipped them was really slick. Koolie worked under the basket and developed a method of hooking his elbow over their center to prevent him from rebounding. Have you ever seen a six-foot-five-inch guy cry during a basketball game? Every time he would try to jump, Koolie "accidentally" hooked him and out-rebounded him something awful. Meanwhile, the other guard, Robert Campbell, (we did have a few normal names, although we pronounced it *Camel*), and I were shooting over their guards from almost mid-court and we couldn't miss. We hit on almost everything we threw at the basket. If I remember correctly, Koolie scored 16 points and I hit 15 for a total of 31 of the 41 we scored that night. Our normal individual average was something like 4 or 5 points per game. Incredible!

~

GOOD friends are hard to come by. And a really true friend can be worth more to you than you may know at the moment. Many years ago I came to realize what a really good friend Koolie has been.

~

MY last year of high school was my best year, ever, in football. Just that year, we had gone from 6-man to 11-man and I, as one of the fastest running backs in our senior class of 31 students, scored two-thirds of the points that our team scored for the entire season. What a thrill! I'll never forget either one of those two touchdowns!

~

MANY years later, while living in Minneapolis, I became good friends with a witty, hard-drinking Irishman named Jack. He and his wife, Opal, lived just across the street and had some of the most hilarious true stories I've ever heard.

One of the few that isn't "R" rated concerned his father, Bert, who played baseball as a young man with one of the local high school teams. Bert had a rather confrontational relationship with one of his male teachers who never missed a chance to needle him. Once, at a game down in Wilmer, Minnesota, Bert, who was the best player on the team and could play any position, was called on to substitute for the catcher, who had been hurt rather badly in a collision at the plate. Of course, Bert didn't even own a protective cup and, of course, never wore one at his regular position at second base. And, of course, the first pitch went right through his glove and, of course, got him right in the "of courses."

The next day, in front of the whole class, the teacher said, "I hear you got hit yesterday, Bert."

"That's right," he answered.

"Where'd you get hit, Bert?" asked the teacher with a devilish grin.

"In Wilmer," replied Bert with a straight face.

~

STEP # 4

Pick a Q-Buddy

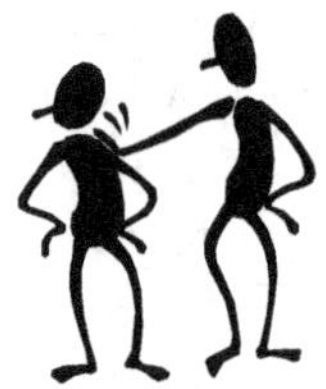

JUST as we rely on each other in team sports to see us through to victory, so, too, will a **Q-Buddy** be vital to the victory over addiction.

If you have a spouse, relative or friend who also wants to quit, choose them for your **Q-Buddy**. Somebody you will listen to and whom you can support in return. It could even be a non-smoker who is close to you. Maybe it's somebody that responded enthusiastically to your **Q-Note**.

♥ Someone you can call when you have that urge for a smoke.

♥ Someone to hang out with, take a walk, watch TV.

♥ Someone to share your sense of uneasiness, your cravings and temptations.

**So, give them a shout and let them help you to
kick this ugly habit.**

Be a **TEAM** - <u>T</u>ogether <u>E</u>veryone <u>A</u>chieves <u>M</u>ore.
Be each other's anchor in the storm.
Be a champion for each other — to each other.

~

*The best way to find yourself
is to lose yourself in the service to others.*
Mahatma Mohandas Karamchand Gandhi

~

CHAPTER 5

Q-DAY EVE

OH, boy! Tomorrow's the big day!

This thought kept going through my mind as I tried to go to sleep in Grandmother and Poppy's house at 1040 N. Kenwood St. in Burbank, California. *Tomorrow, I begin my studies at Glendale College.*

But the events leading up to this day had a profound effect on my life.

~

WHEN we entered WW II, Poppy decided that the automobile business was over, at least for the duration. So, being the patriot that he was, he sold his dealership and moved to Akron, Ohio, to go to work at the Goodyear plant. Being far too old to serve in the military, he became an inspector there and quickly rose to department head. He was absolutely correct about the new car business being defunct, but he badly miscalculated in selling his dealership. I remember the auction where he sold new Fords for as little as $200, and nearly-new used cars for $50 to $100. Those same automobiles would bring thousands of dollars in a very short time as the auto industry switched over to building tanks, planes and guns.

But Poppy never looked back. He and Uncle Bernard, who had made the move before them, soon became totally involved, often times working two shifts straight. Uncle Bernard received a beautifully engraved award from Goodyear in recognition of his invention of the process for welding the wheels used in the fighter planes built by Grumman, Vought-Sikorsky, etc. If the wheels, which had a high content of magnesium, came out of the presses with any flaw they were simply discarded.

Uncle Bernard's process saved untold thousands of dollars and, more importantly, saved raw material sorely needed for our war effort. After the war, he eventually wound up his exceptional career as an executive in the jet engine division of GE Corporation.

Not long after the war's outbreak, my Dad abandoned us. For more than two years, we had no idea where he was or if he was even alive. Uncle John, (who had finally "killed" Madren), flew in one day in his Navion and picked me up from school to go look for him. What a hero I was that day. Here comes this sleek plane, which resembled a smaller Bell P-39 Airacobra, landing in the field right next to our football field, (the one that had the grandstand behind which I "taught Koolie how to smoke.")

Uncle John had become one of the world's best-known professional magicians, ranking right up there with Blackstone, Thurston and Dante. He was under contract with one of the major studios in Hollywood, altogether acting in over 40 films, and starred in the last few *Falcon* detective series. He is one of, if not the best, stage performers I have ever seen, in any venue, with his natural charm and his devastating good looks. He went on to carry his magic show, *Magicarama,* around the world, entertaining the troops during the war and continuing long afterward, receiving rave reviews in almost every language. When he finally returned home, the entire family followed him and settled in California.

He continued performing and giving lectures for a long time, and, in August of 2012, he celebrated his 101st birthday by performing at Hollywood's *Magic Castle.* He died the next year at 102. May he rest in peace.

~

IN my mid-teens, after not knowing where my father was half the time, my parents finally divorced. Afterwards, my mother took over the job of sole support for us three boys. Many mornings I would awaken at 5:00 a.m. to one of the Greyhound drivers, Art or Frank, blowing the horn for Mom. She rode the bus to Cincinnati, about 30 miles away, where she would then take the streetcar to Bethesda Hospital on Reading Road and work for two straight shifts, take the streetcar to catch the bus back to Harrison where she fed us, washed our clothes, slept for maybe three or four hours and then reversed the entire process. She did this seven days a week for over three years. The only time she would take off was to attend my games. She rarely missed one. My mother was a saint.

~

Human beings are the only creatures that allow
their children to come back home.
Bill Cosby

~

AND SO, here I was, ready to begin college. What should I study? What did I want to do? Law? Medicine? I ruled out engineering since I had flunked both Algebra and Plane Geometry. And then I ruled out Medicine since I almost flunked Biology. Back then, lawyers weren't held in the same high esteem that they enjoy today, so that was out. But I had done very well with three years of Spanish and decided to take a fourth year of it, even though I didn't think I wanted to become a Spaniard. In addition, I opted for Public Speaking 101, Social Studies and several music courses as well as Drama. I sang in the A Cappella Choir and the Male Octet which performed for several churches and other schools.

It was while four of us were returning from one such engagement, being chauffeured by our accompanist, Betty, that we discovered we had the makings of a great quartet. And so we began haunting bars where we found that, just by sitting unobtrusively in a booth and starting to sing quietly, we soon had someone passing a tray and collecting no small amount of money. This was good.

We entered the Fox West Coast Talent Contest, winning at the first few levels and finally appearing for the district finals at the El Portal Theater in North Hollywood. We lost to Harry Capps, a really talented fellow who stood on one hand, tap danced on a platform over his head while playing the trumpet. We found out that he had packed the first few rows (right next to the applause meter) with all his friends and relatives who raised holy heck ("hell" having not yet been discovered on college campuses), sending the meter off the scale when his vote came up. Here is where I decided that it's not whether you win or lose, it's how you cheat the game that counts. Of course, I outgrew that soon enough, but it was a bitter pill to swallow. We were, however, invited to perform for the Grand Finals as an opening act at Grauman's Chinese Theater in Hollywood. A great thrill!

~

A PATTERN was beginning to emerge in my life that took me many years to recognize. Without realizing it, I was being prepared for the mission that drives me today. I believe that every person has it within him or her to achieve great things. It just needs to be recognized. Once recognized, one must put on the blinders and plow straight ahead towards that ideal. Just think what you have the opportunity to do right now.

By showing everyone that YOU can conquer your addiction, you can motivate countless others to follow your example!

~

For a man to conquer himself
is the first and noblest of all victories.
PLATO

~

STEP # 5

Q-Day Eve

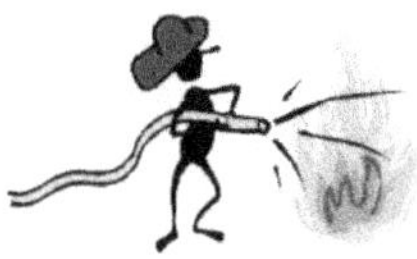

TODAY, the evening before you quit, we **prepare for tomorrow** and all the smoke-free tomorrows to come.

Spend today **smoking up a storm!** Unless you've been cutting down (which is very difficult to do), you need to overload your system with the drug, thereby giving you a head start for tomorrow. You'll wake up with an awful, dirty brown taste in your mouth, not wanting a cigarette till noon. It will help you through the first few hours.

While this is a very short step, it's just as important as all the rest of them. It's like if you leave any one number out of a phone number, you'll never reach the person you want to talk to . . . (A preposition is something you should never end a sentence with . . .)

Also, just before you hit the sack:

- Throw away the last of your cigarettes,
- Get rid of your ashtrays, but —
- **Keep your lighter.** Interesting, right? I'll tell you why in Step # 6.

~

You were born to win,
but to be the winner you were born to be,
*you have to **plan** to win and **prepare** to win.*
Then and only then can you expect to win.
"Born to Win"
Zig Ziglar

~

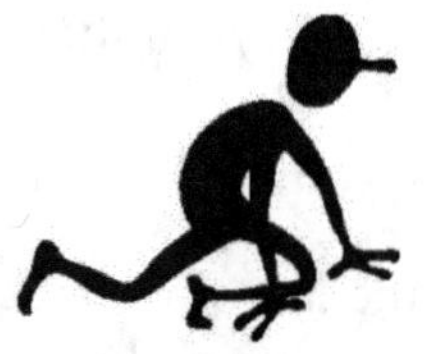

Get Ready!

Get Set! . . .

CHAPTER 6

Q-DAY!

ON the sixth of June 1944, D-Day, tens of thousands of American soldiers and their allies stormed the beaches at Normandy to mark the beginning of the end to the madness that was WW II. My summer vacation had just begun, between the eighth grade and my first year of high school. Some of my recollections of the war:

- Paper drives;
- Searching for scrap metal, especially aluminum;
- "A","B", and "C" stickers on windshields depicting the type of gasoline allotment the driver was entitled to, "A" being the best;
- A nationwide speed limit of 35 mph;
- Books of ration stamps for meat and sugar, among other things;
- War Bonds and books of stamps that, when filled by purchasing enough at 25 or 50 cents, could be traded for a War Bond whose value at purchase was $18.75, but would be redeemed at some date in the future for $25.00;
- Mom saving cups of grease to be turned in for part of the ingredients of nitro-glycerin;
- Giant posters of Uncle Sam looking sternly right at you and saying, "I Need YOU!"
- Signs saying "Loose Lips Sink Ships;"
- War movies with John Wayne, Ward Bond, Errol Flynn, Clark Gable, Lana Turner, Betty Grable, Betty Hutton and many, many others;

♬ - Bob Hope on USO tours entertaining the troops, with Francis Langford and Jerry Colona, often right behind the lines;

♬ - Fox Movietone News at the little movie theater on Harrison Avenue showing our boys in action;

♬ - Concession food at the movies: popcorn was 10 cents, 15 cents with butter, which, during the war, became margarine into which you had to mix the powdered color; a coke was five cents for six ounces, but you got "Twice as much for a nickel, too . . ." with Pepsi;

♬ - Gasoline, when you could get it, was 15 to 20 cents per gallon;

♬ - Cigarettes, when you could get them, were 20 cents a pack except for Raleighs, which actually gave you three cents change from a quarter wrapped right in the outer cellophane if you bought them from a machine.

And, oh, the Patriotic songs:

♪ -"Any Bonds Today . . ."

♫ - "Praise The Lord and Pass the Ammunition."

♪ - "Comin' In On A Wing And A Prayer . . ."

♫ - "There'll Be Blue Birds Over, The White Cliffs Of Dover . . ." — *(So, watch out!)*

There was never any doubt in anyone's mind that we were going to prevail, and that "When the lights go on again, all over the world . . ." things would return to normal — my Dad would come home and live with us, and Poppy and Grandmother and Uncle Bernard would come back and things would be right again.

Of course, it didn't happen. Not all of it.

~

AFTER my one year of college, where I won election as freshman class president on a platform of "Free Love and Beer in Every Drinking Fountain," (I didn't deliver or get either one), I returned to Ohio to live with my mother and brothers while working in a factory in Connersville, Indiana, making Philco refrigerators. This one year of my personal history could be sufficient grist for several chapters. Suffice it to say that I was not the sharpest tool in the shed at this point in my life, and I had a lot of maturing to do. Oh, nothing illegal, or at least nothing of a felonious nature, and nothing mean to my family or anything like that. It was simply a period of wasted time, wasted effort and wasted opportunity. Maybe another time, another book.

And then came the "Greetings" from the President of the United States, pleading with me to come help him with the Korean thing! Since I had missed some Naval Reserve meetings when I left North Hollywood without even saying goodbye to my chief, he became offended and told the draft board about it and, hence, the letter from President Truman.

I volunteered for immediate induction and reported to Fort Ord, California, and was quickly sent to Camp Roberts, California. Because of my previous service in the U.S. Navy, I entered at one grade higher as an E-2 (squad leader and no K.P.), and, because there was a war going on in Korea, I only did six weeks of basic training. I had scored very well on my testing at Ft. Ord, especially on the Morse Code aptitude test, and went into Intermediate Speed Radio Operators School at Camp Roberts. From there, after a short stint as an instructor, I went on to Leadership School, graduating with sergeant stripes and headed for Ft. Benning, Georgia, and Infantry Officer's Candidate School, aka *Benning's School for Boys* —

"Here lie the bones of Lt. Jones,
a graduate of this institution.
He died last night, in his first fire-fight,
using the school solution."
(Carved on a desk in one of the classrooms.)

~

Oh, the fun, the adventure, the endless hours of harassment and humiliation, the TAC Officers, the Blue Beatles, the hopelessness and despair. One young candidate crawled under the next barracks and ended his life by eating his M-1. Somehow I survived and was graduated, an officer and a gentleman by act of congress, somewhere in the middle of my class.

Due to being enrolled in one school after another, including Infantry Officers Communication School, Airborne training, etc., I spent 24 months of my 30-month total in school and never got to Korea. Praise God! There's another book here, as well, and maybe I'll write it someday. I would have to tell the whole story of how, on my 21st birthday, I tried in vain to get some bartender, any bartender, to check my I.D. They carried me back to the barracks, totally unchecked.

~

WHAT in the world, you may well ask, does all this have to do with **Q-Day**? Simple!

It's Your **LIBERATION DAY!**
The First Day of your Smoke-Free-Forever Life!

While I flailed around trying to find myself in my early manhood, there were habits that I had formed that would someday be broken, (the bad ones), and eventually replaced with — a code of living that has brought me peace of mind and a feeling of being **OK** with myself.

YOU are now on the threshold of that same type of freedom.

Stay tuned for the BIG SECRETS of —

QUITTING WITHOUT CLIMBING THE WALLS.

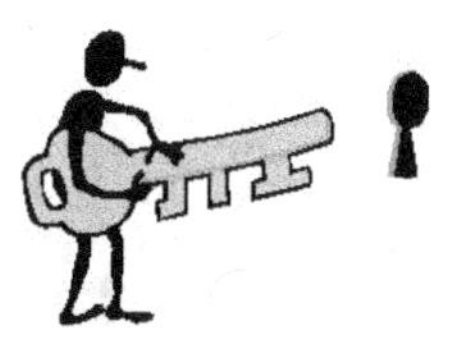

> # STEP # 6
>
> ## Q-Day!

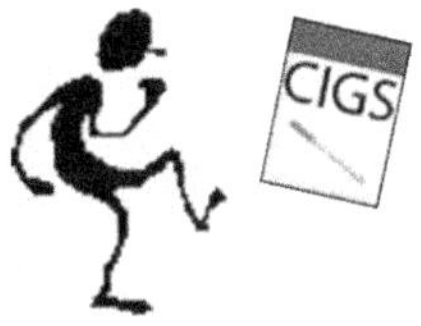

TIME TO KILL THE URGE!

INITIALLY, you must **stay away** from anything that in the past made you want a cigarette, like:

~ coffee, and perhaps

~ alcohol, or

~ whatever else it might be for you..

This will only be for a few days — I promise.

> ## BIG SECRET - PART I
>
> ### DEEP and RAPID BREATHING

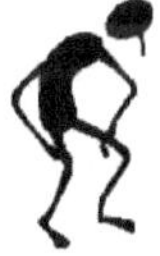

Also known as HYPERVENTILATION. (**Check with your doctor** if this step is ok for you). Until you get used to this, you might want to sit down while doing it or you may find yourself flat on your back looking up at the ceiling. **You'll be absolutely amazed** at how effective this is!

> ## BIG SECRET - PART II
>
> ### KEEP YOUR LIGHTER

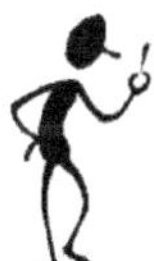

Every time you feel the monkey squeezing you, **flick your lighter while you do some deep breathing,** and watch the urge to strangle the little old lady sitting next to you completely disappear. It works! It **really** works!

Whenever anyone around you is starting to light up, **whip out your lighter** and light it for them while you tell them: "I'm doing this for me, not for you."

What you're doing with these "secrets" is satisfying two urges at once:

1 - The chemical one, by delivering an over-abundance of oxygen that the nicotine depletes to your respiratory system, and

2 - The mechanical one, which keeps your hands busy doing a familiar chore.

I kept my lighter for almost five years before I discovered that, after I had forgotten it one morning, I didn't need it any more.

The urges will become fewer and farther between until, one day, you'll realize you're free, totally free!

In the next chapter we'll discover some ways to minimize the temptations and a lot of other good stuff.

Read On!

~

Be sure that when your ship comes in, you're not at the airport.
A. Nonymous

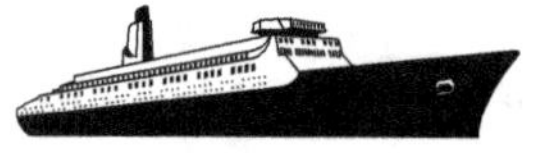

~

CHAPTER 7

NEVER SMOKE AGAIN!

THEY say that opportunity never knocks twice. Baloney! If that were true, I would still be working in the paint department getting steel shells ready to be painted and turned into Philco fridges. Our problem, usually, is that we often fail to recognize the knock. It's almost like we're waiting for a special code — knock knock *(pause) knock (pause)* knock knock knock — and so on. Most of us are waiting for the doorbell to ring and, when we open it, find a TV crew and all kinds of people with flowers yelling:

> *"Congratulations! You've just won first prize!*
> *ONE week paid vacation to Keokuk, Iowa!"*
> *("Second prize - TWO weeks in Keokuk!!")*

~

THERE are three kinds of people;
    ~ Those who make things happen,
    ~ Those who watch things happen, and
    ~ Those who sit around and say, "What happened?"

THIS reminds me — There are another 'three kinds of people':
    ~ Those who are good at math and
    ~ Those who are not.

~

MY little brothers are two distinctly different examples of the "make-things-happen" category. Robert, the one who got me the whipping of my life just because I offered him his first nicotine taste, went all the way through high school in Harrison, four years of college graduating Phi Beta Kappa from Berkley, and topped it all off with a doctor of "philosophyship" from "Haavaad," in Cambridge, Mass. None of this education seems to have hurt him very much, and he retired as a highly respected professor of Political Science at a prestigious midwestern college. When he was once asked what kind of doctor he was, he replied, "I'm the kind that doesn't do anybody any good." I'm sure there are those on both extremes of the political spectrum who would agree with him, but I happen to think he's pretty smart. A whole lot more in tune with the world and what's happening in it than a lot of his colleagues. He was very active in the effort to obtain the release of a former instructor who had been imprisoned for several years in Egypt for the "crime" of having politically incorrect material advocating democracy. I'm very proud of my brother Robert.

Freddie, my youngest brother, who now prefers to be called either Fred, or "One Hundred Eighty Pounds of Stompin' Romance," is a real, honest-to-goodness Hollywood producer. He started out in the animation department at Disney Studios (at my prompting, which he still doesn't remember) in Burbank, went to Hanna-Barbera for a while, and then struck out on his own, doing some 70+% of the animation for the original Sesame Street. Before he left Disney, he invited me to be a part of the production of *Sleeping Beauty*.

I was very excited about this chance and arrived at the studio *as nervous as a guy sittin' in a sports car surrounded by tall dogs.* Fred brought me into the room where all these weird looking people were sitting on high chairs bent over drawings of cartoon characters. The more I looked, the more they started to resemble tall dogs.

"Are you ready to become a part of history?" he beamed.

"I certainly am," I beamed back.

"Good," he re-beamed, "Take this pen and carefully draw a line on the horse's tail, from here to here," indicating a space about one inch long. Even though I felt nervous, I knew that I would calm down as I became more accustomed to the tremendous tension I felt, what with all the glances I got from these cartoonists, none of whom were beaming, and the desire to make my youngest brother proud of me, who also wasn't beaming at the moment. He, too, felt my tension.

I took the pen firmly in hand and stroked the line as sure as an arrow flying straight and true to its target.

"There, how does it feel to be immortalized?" he asked, with a beam back.

"That's all?" I half-beamed.

"That's it!" he replied, beaming even brighter.

And so, my immortality is there for all to see, on the rear end of Prince Charming's horse — IF you happen to be looking in the exact right spot during that 180,000,000th of a second. (I noticed that I didn't receive a credit at the end of the picture.)

Today, Fred is doing quite well, working on a live action feature film which he has written and is both directing and producing. 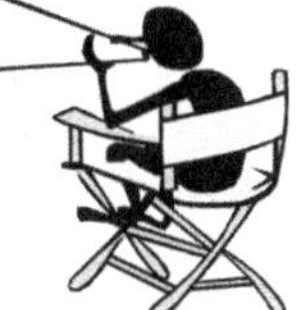

He is still beaming.

~

KOOLIE also deserves mention for his successes. He, too, served his country, staying in the U.S. Navy for a full hitch, then going on to graduate from Ohio State Veterinary School. He stayed in Harrison until his retirement and established a practice which was one of the best in the tri-state area.

He once confided to me that he had considered getting an additional degree in Taxidermy.

"Either way," he said, "you get your dog back."

Author's note: One of the most difficult things I have ever had to do was to read a eulogy at Bill's funeral, March 17, 2011. May he rest in peace. Miss you so much, Koolie, My Friend.

~

TOP 10 REASONS WHY
YOU'LL NEVER SMOKE AGAIN

10. You've never smoked in the first place. Everyone's been lying.

9. You're not a teenager anymore, so now it's legal.

8. You're tired of mooches "borrowing" cigarettes.

7. The smoking areas are full of smokers.

6. Your mother-in-law said you'd never be able to quit.

5. Jumping from a really high building is quicker.

4. The cost of cigarettes is taking away from your gambling addiction.

3. You'll cut your exposure time by sleeping 16 hours a day.

2. You'll smell a lot better.

1. Since you smell so much better, your mate won't be able to keep their hands off you.

Personally, I believe you will not start again for the simple reason that, having followed the first six steps, you arc now prepared for Step # 7.

~

The key to WILL power is WANT-power.
*People who **want** something badly enough*
*can usually find the **will** power to achieve it!*
Anonymous

~

> # STEP # 7
>
> ## Never Smoke Again!

WELL, duh! If I never smoke again, of *course,* I'll have quit. This isn't as silly as it sounds.

Most people who fail, do so because they haven't prepared themselves **psychologically.** They put out a cigarette and say to themselves, *That's it! I quit!* They may even throw away a few remaining in the pack — but it's just an impulse, nothing more. As soon as the nicotine craving returns, it's all over. The addiction is just too strong.

**Most experts agree that nicotine is
far harder to kick than heroin.**

I suspect one reason is that cigarettes are still legal for adults and, therefore, carry at least a semblance of respectability. But even that is slowly disappearing.

Chances are, you started at a very young age. Statistics say that 90% of smokers begin before the age of 20. That's when you were either rebelling or trying to "fit in."

Guess what — it's way past the time to end the rebellion, and you're finding that you don't fit in where it counts anymore.

Avoid situations which will **TRIGGER your craving.** Take a few days off from your normal routine. Things like:

MORNING COFFEE – "No, no! I'll die if I don't have my coffee!" No, you won't; you will live! And besides, it's very temporary — a few days at most.

ALCOHOL — You can do it! It's so worth it!

ANYTHING ELSE that makes you want to smoke.

Just for a few days!

Bite the bullet.

Deep breathe!

Flick your "bic"!

YOU. ARE. STRONGER. NOW!!!!!

~

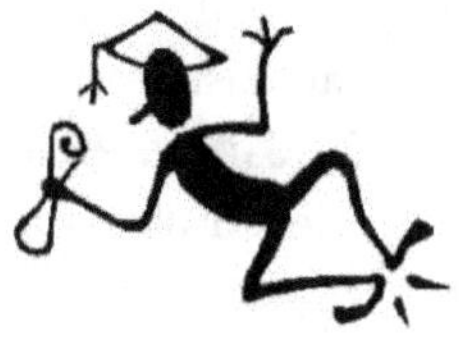

CHAPTER 8

LIFE WITHOUT THE MONKEY

NOW that you've successfully kicked the monkey off your back, let's talk seriously about keeping him off.

There's an old saying that "experience is the best teacher." This is only true up to a point.

> *Experience is the best teacher*
> **as long as** *it's someone else's experience.*

Why should we make mistakes that others have made, if they're willing to share their experience with us, mentor us and guide us? Usually, the only thing that keeps anyone from doing this is pride.

"I already know that."
"You can't tell me anything new."

Know anyone like that? It wouldn't be you, would it? Let's assume it isn't and give you the benefit of my several flawed attempts at quitting.

~

WHEN I was doing my television show in Minneapolis, I was a fairly well-known personality. The day of the taping of my first "Special" for WCCO-TV, the local CBS affiliate, I was taking congratulations after the taping from one and all, and generally feeling pretty self-important. I had noticed a couple of well-dressed gentlemen standing off to one side, but didn't pay any particular attention to them, as I didn't want to miss one pat on the back or "Well done." Soon, my producer, Fred King, came up to me and said he wanted to introduce me to someone. I was on a roll, my glib responses had been rolling off my tongue with ease and, as I approached the two gentlemen that I had noticed before, I was prepared to receive more of the same laudatory praises. All in the same instant, I stuck out my hand, recognized the taller of the two, just as Fred was saying, "Mel, I'd like you to meet Ed Ames."

For you youngsters, Ed Ames was the co-star of the old Davy Crockett TV series and played "Mingo," Crockett's faithful Indian companion. Furthermore, he was a superstar long before this, as one of the world-famous Ames Brothers Trio ("The Naughty Lady of Shady Lane," "Cab Driver,") and he had long been one of my show biz idols.

So, what did I say to him, me, the guy who had just knocked 'em dead with a local TV show, the guy who was feeling mighty good about himself, so self-assured, the big "star" who everyone was patting on the back and congratulating? I looked up into his face from my full 5-ft, 7-inch height, which seemed at least four feet below him, and said in total awe,

"Ed Ames! . . . Gee Whiz!"

Never in my life have I been so tongue-tied! Since then, I've entertained royalty and heads of state with flawless aplomb, but I'll always remember my faithful producer, "Jolly Tall" Fred King, who also served as my "Hugh Downs," making several references to me in subsequent shows as "The ever-eloquent Mel Calvert."

~

I DID several long engagements at the top night spots in town and had a reputation for "putting rear-ends on the seats." After hours, we in the "show biz" field would gather at one of the all-night restaurants where we would make merry, telling jokes and tall tales to each other about how our careers were "really taking off," and just generally gossiping like a bunch of old ladies. It was quite usual for me to get home as the sun was coming up.

One particular night, the subject of smoking came up and someone bet that none of us could quit. Always being one to accept a challenge, I said I could quit anytime I wanted to.

Little by little, we bantered back and forth until we came up with a money challenge. Everyone would put in twenty bucks, and, at the end of 90 days, those who still hadn't smoked would divide up the pot. Honor system. Since there were only five or six of us there that evening, we set a deadline of some three or four days to get as many in as we could and ended up with a total of ten people willing to do it. We all reasoned that the least that would happen if we all quit would be that we'd get our money back.

In a very few days, several dropped out — then a couple more — until there were only two of us who then divided up the $200. Everyone was satisfied that nobody had cheated. But, just to prove my original point that I could quit anytime I wanted to, and that I didn't need a bet to do it, I stayed off for another 30 days, just for good measure.

Then I said to myself, *Well, I've proved I can do it and that's good enough for me. Now, I'm ready for a smoke.*

Several months passed until, one day, I got to thinking about how much better the food had tasted when I was off, and how much easier it was to breathe, how I smelled better and how I generally just felt better. So, I decided it was time to quit for good. This time it only lasted for a month, and the realization hit me — **I had a monkey on my back.**

But, instead of getting angry about it, I resigned myself to being a smoker for the rest of my life and really didn't give it a lot more thought.

Not, that is, until my famous Uncle John gave me enough grief that I decided it wasn't worth it to continue taking his constant, good-natured needling. And so, as a concession to him, which was totally the wrong reason, I quit again.

Don't just quit for somebody else. Do it for you.

NO one else is nearly as affected by this legal poison as you. Certainly, it's good that your family, especially your defenseless children, will benefit from your quitting. Not only in the short term, but they'll also benefit for the many more years they will have *you* around to love.

In the final analysis, **you must do it, first and foremost, for yourself.** Only then will others reap the benefits.

~

EIGHTEEN months after quitting *for* my uncle, I started again . . . *because* of him. We're both strong personalities and we were constantly clashing over the pettiest of things. One clash was not so petty, and the ensuing falling-out was all I needed to invite the monkey back. *I'll bring you back just so my uncle can see what a stubborn person he is,* I said to the monkey. *Come on, hop on! Let's show him he can't tell* **me** *what to do!*

Not only was that stupid, but also the mere fact of letting someone else get to me was the biggest stupidity of all. Fortunately, it didn't take me very long to realize that. And so, after a lot of trial and error, and a lot of research, I came up with the seven steps in just about the same form in which they remain today as the **"7 Steps To Life."**

~

ARE there other methods available? Sure. They almost all cost money, sometimes month after month after month. There's the drug, Chantix™, with horrible side effects. Who wants that? Some of the most popular is the patch; another is nicotine gum. And now, nicotine toothpicks. More bad actors just trying to cash in on your addiction.

I've tried them at one time or another. But the nicotine patch, gum and toothpicks are *designed* to fail.

Why?

Because they simply change the point of the drug introduction from one place on your body to another.

~

THAT would be like saying to an alcoholic, "We're going to take away your bottle and hook you up to an alcohol IV."

I can just hear the answer — "Cool!"

~

OR, as the judge says sternly to the drunk, "You've been brought in here for drinking!"

The drunk hiccups and slurs, "Fine, your Honor, let's get started!"

~

HOW long will it take — and when will you know for sure — that the monkey is gone?

For many months after my final decision to quit, I had a recurring nightmare. In my dream, I would find myself smoking a cigarette. When the realization of what I was doing hit me, I experienced a terrible feeling of remorse.

"Oh, no! What am I doing? I was doing so well. Why did I do this?" The feeling of sadness, almost a sickness, that I experienced is impossible to put into words.

By the same token, when I awoke and realized it was only a dream, the feeling of euphoria almost made the horror of the nightmare worthwhile.

The monkey was gone for good!

~

I once dreamed I was eating a 15-pound marshmallow.
When I woke up, my pillow was gone!
Anonny Muss

~

WHAT YOU HAVE TO LOOK FORWARD TO
WITHOUT THE MONKEY

· Within **20 minutes**, after putting out your last cigarette, blood pressure and pulse rate return to normal.

· Within **three hours**, "smoker's breath" disappears. The carbon monoxide level in blood drops and the oxygen level returns to normal

· Within **24 hours**, chance of heart attack decreases.

· Within **two days**, nerve endings start to regroup, and the ability to taste and smell improves.

· After **three days**, breathing is easier.

· Within **two to three months**, circulation improves; walking becomes easier; lung capacity increases up to 30%.

· **One to nine months** after your last cigarette, sinus congestion and shortness of breath decrease; cilia that sweeps debris from your lungs grow back; energy increases!

· Within **one year**, the excess risk of coronary heart disease is half that of a smoker's.

· Heart attack risk drops to near normal within **two years**.

· Within **five years**, lung cancer death rate for the average former pack-a-day smoker decreases by almost half. Stroke is reduced; risk of mouth, throat and esophageal cancer is half that of a smoker's.

· Within **10 years**, lung cancer death rate is similar to that of a person who does not smoke; the pre-cancerous cells are replaced.

· And, finally, within **15 years**, the risk of coronary heart disease is the same as a person who has never smoked.

Any Questions?

Please follow each and every step faithfully, to the letter.
The wonderful truth is — if you follow ALL the steps,
you **will** win, and
the monkey **will** lose.

DON'T SKIP A STEP!!

This program can be compared to a recipe for a cake. Don't decide that you're only going to do certain steps and leave out others.

If you leave out the eggs in a cake recipe, it ain't cake. Or it sure won't taste nearly as good.

Same here. **Each step is absolutely vital.** It builds upon the prior step.

So, for your sake and the sake of the friends and loved ones cheering for you, **stick to the program,** and you, too, will enjoy the smoke-free life that my family and I have enjoyed for almost forty years.

I know you can do it!

You know you can do it!

JUST GO FOR IT!

~

*If you think you can or you think you can't —
you're right.*
Henry Ford

~

~

Today, over 1300 people will stop smoking in America.
Their funerals will be held this week.

~

CHAPTER 9

PREPARE TO WIN!

"7 STEPS TO LIFE" REVIEW

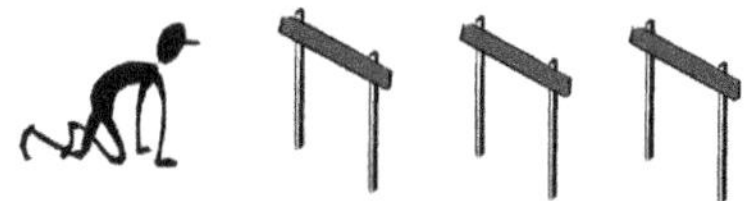

1 – ADMIT YOU'RE AN ADDICT
"MIRROR, MIRROR, ON THE WALL"

Face the mirror. Admit to yourself that you're an addict. It does no good whatsoever to admit it to anyone else until you admit it to yourself

---

2 – PICK YOUR Q-DAY
GO GET YOUR CALENDAR

This is another crucial part to the mental preparation.
By making your **Quit Day** somewhere in the near future, that day when you say goodbye to your addiction, you can relax a little. "I **am** going to do it!" You're facing the inevitable, but not right this minute. You're giving yourself time to prepare. This is so very important.

---

3 – TELL THE WORLD!
GET ON 'STAGE'!   USE YOUR PHONE & EMAIL

"Come on, be real." How many of us want to admit that we can't do something. Especially if we tell everyone that **we are going to do it!** The importance of this step can't be over-stressed. It will give you a lot more stamina to realize that, if you don't quit, you're not only letting yourself down, but also a lot of people who care about you and many who depend on you for their well-being.

4 – PICK A Q-BUDDY
KNOW WHO YOUR REAL FRIENDS ARE

Isn't it a lot more enjoyable to experience a good movie, TV show or concert *with* someone — rather than alone? Of course, it is! Therefore, a good friend or loved one who is there for you when you feel weak, your **Q-Buddy**, is equally good. If you are mates and both quitting — Hallelujah!

5 – Q-DAY EVE
START A FIRE TO PUT OUT A FIRE!

Preparing for the big day by an overindulgence in nicotine the night before may seem a bit extreme, but the logic is clear. By loading up on the drug the night before, you'll get a head start when you wake up. A cigarette is the last thing you'll want.

Also, **get rid of your remaining cigarettes** and **dispose of your ashtrays.** Your house should be smoke-free from now on. Let house visitors know that, from this day on, they go outside to smoke.

6 – Q-DAY!
KICK SOME BUTTS – KILL THE URGE!

Deep and rapid breathing at the **first** sign of craving. Remember Lamaze classes? A lot like that.

Flick your lighter. There's really no way to describe how effective this is until you do it. But do it right!

7 – NEVER SMOKE AGAIN!
AVOID YOUR PERSONAL SMOKING TRIGGERS

No coffee for several days or more, **no alcohol** for the same amount of time. **Anything that triggers your craving** should be avoided for as long as it takes to get your withdrawals under control, usually no more than a few days. This includes any situation that is conducive to a **"sociable" smoke.** Avoid them, too. If you've never tried to quit before, you'll be amazed just how quickly the cravings subside.

A **CAUTION**, however, is in order.

"Subside" doesn't mean "Goes Away Completely."
An addict's an addict . . .

It took me several weeks before I stopped **thinking** about smoking, and even then, a freshly lit cigarette could make me drool, (almost), even though the cravings had all but disappeared. My challenge was all the bigger since I quit while I was still appearing in night clubs where everybody smoked.

What's more, I had a routine in my magic act that had to have a cigarette to be effective. It started with several quick dove "appearances" after which I set them on top of a cage. Then I borrowed a lit cigarette from someone in the audience (at that time, smoking was still allowed in public indoor places). Next, after a few manipulations, I vanish the lit cigarette into my fist and open my hand to show it's gone. I look over at the doves sitting on the cage and do a double take. I then walk over to the cage, pick up a bird and "appear" to pull the cigarette out of the dove's rear end!

It was always good for a laugh and I was still able to quit smoking completely even though I took several puffs from the cigarette during the hand manipulations. I never inhaled.

But even that soon became nasty to me, so I was very relieved when we finally gave up the act and ate the doves. (OF COURSE, we didn't!)

~

Each of us was born with wings and has the ability
to go farther than we ever thought possible
and to do things beyond our wildest imagination.
Barbara Stanny

~

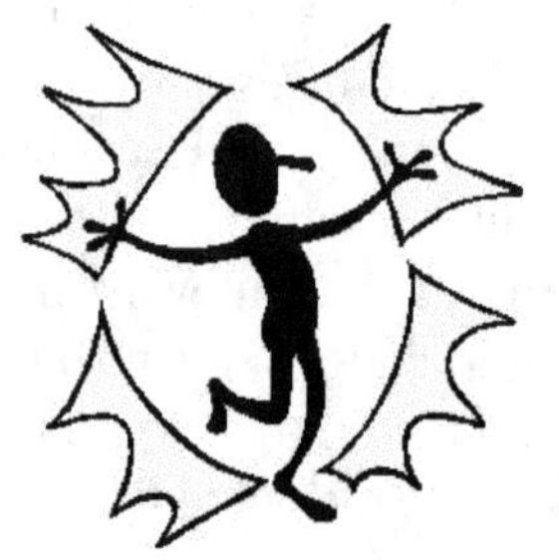

SOURCES

THE research for this book and for the "7 Steps To Life" smoking cessation program was compiled from the author's own personal experience, surveys of smokers throughout the country and scientific data from government agencies.

We gratefully acknowledge the following associations for their research. Without their making it available to the general public, this book would not have been possible.

> The American Cancer Society
> The American Heart Association
> The American Lung Association
> The Centers for Disease Control (CDC)
> U.S. Department of Health and Human Services
> National Center for Health Statistics
> National Center for Injury Prevention and Control

TESTIMONIALS & REVIEWS

7 Steps to Life Smoking Cessation Program and the book,
How I Quit Smoking and Lived To Tell About It

"Although I quit smoking some thirty years ago, this was fun to read. Mel's methods are safe, effective and based on sound principles. This is one of the best and most entertaining books I have read in months. I highly recommend the book and his humor."
— Burt Prelutsky, TV Script Writer: MASH, The Bob Newhart Show, Mary Tyler Moore and many others.

* * *

"What I like so much about this book and the method it describes is its total natural approach. One wants to say, 'This is so logical that it's not funny.' But he makes it funny, and the timing couldn't be better. Enjoy."
—Jonathan Silver, MD, Syndicated columnist and talk show host

* * *

"Here's a guy after my own heart. Tells it like it is . . . and if you don't laugh while you're reading it, it went over your head. Read it again while you're standing up!"
—Joe Franklin, Holder of the Guinness Book of Records for the longest syndicated talk show in history

* * *

"This method, '7 steps to Life,' is medically safe and very effective in breaking the nicotine addiction. If one follows each of the *7 steps* to the letter, he or she will never want to smoke again."
— Dr. Wm. Kuhlmann, Cincinnati, OH

* * *

"I lost my husband, his parents and his two brothers. His sister has emphysema and is on oxygen. All of this because of smoking cigarettes. They all wanted to quit but couldn't. If only they had known about *7 Steps.*
— L. Reilly, Lake City, FL

* * *

"I 'quit' dozens of times and always went back — until I found your system. Thank you so much for giving me a few more years and in much better health. My cough is gone, and I have so much more energy. Thanks again!"
—J. Hahn, Los Angeles, CA.

* * *

"Dear Mr. Calvert, I wish to thank you for your help in getting my husband off cigarettes. He was smoking 2 packs a day and would not even look at any quit smoking stuff. I worked with him, using your system and I will tell anyone that it works. He has been off for over 90 days now and says he doesn't miss it at all."
— D. Gilchrist, Tempe, AZ

* * *

"I was a three-pack-a-day smoker for over thirty years, and at today's prices, I've been watching over $3,000 a year go up in smoke! But the real important point is that I've been watching myself die slowly! Where were you over 10 years ago when I last tried to quit? Today, thanks to *7 Steps to Life,* marks my 11th week as a non-smoker. . . . I feel much better and I feel relieved. No more monkey on my back! "
— Alberto. I. Izquierdo, Jacksonville, FL

* * *

"I want to say 'Thank you' in so many ways. How do I start? I've been a smoker for 52 years and have tried the gum, the patch, a well-known prescription drug and you name it. I never lasted more than 8 days. Today marks my 31st day on '7 Steps to Life.' I'm home free! Thank you, thank you!"
— Stephen Powers, Jacksonville, FL

* * *

"There is nothing quite like genuine, tickle-the-funny-bone humor to help people learn about serious subjects and inspire them to change. This is Mel Calvert's amazingly successful approach to the deadly addiction of smoking and a timeless guide to — finally — kicking the habit."
— Joan Swirsky, Journalist and Author

* * *

"We were also very impressed with Mr. Calvert's 'Natural approach.' The only way this system could possibly fail is if the user fails to do the relatively easy but very effective steps."
— Cesar E. Ceballos, MD, FAAOS
   Board Certified Orthopaedic Surgeon
   and Sports Medicine Specialist
   Miami, Florida.   www.orthomiami.com

* * *

"I enthusiastically recommend my old (and I do mean 'old') friend's method of Quitting Smoking. The reason that he is old is due entirely to his quitting that nasty habit he once had all those many years ago!"
— Albert L. Weintraub, Author, *Truth, Lies and Legacy*

* * *

"After 15+ years of smoking a pack a day, I came across this book by speaking with the author Mel Calvert, and I truly think that it was meant to be. I have been wanting to cut out this nasty habit for a while, but procrastination always won. That is until I read about the 7 Steps to Life Quit Smoking Program, which was a quick read and full of real-life helpful tips to kick this horrible and deadly habit. Thank you for helping me improve my lifestyle!
— Charles Granados, FL

END NOTE

IT'S important to me to inject just a thought about **worry**. There have been all kinds of "philosofizations" (it's my word and I am standing by it!) about the subject. How often have you heard the most prominent one —

"DON'T WORRY!"

That is total nonsense — and I will prove it. Again, this is from my own, considerable experience:

WORRY IS VITALLY IMPORTANT!

Fully 90% of the things I worry about

NEVER HAPPENS!

So there!

Worry all you want to. **IT WORKS!**

— Mel

www.AuthorsSymposium.com
mel@AuthorsSymposium.com

~

ABOUT THE AUTHOR

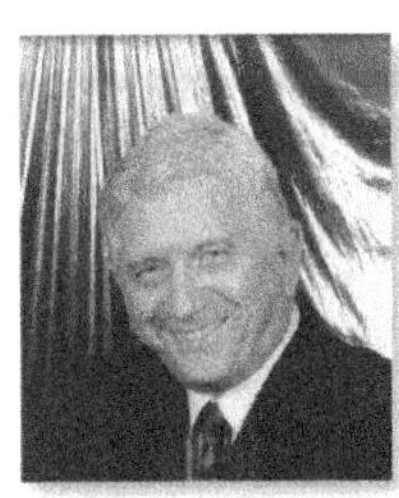

MEL CALVERT has many years of professional communication experience, spanning from an early position in the U.S. Army as a Communications Officer to later becoming a political campaign communications director.

Calvert, together with his wife, Sunny, are a very well-known premier music, magic and comedy show. They have performed for royalty and other heads of state all over the world. They are featured on the album, *Here's a Little Sunshine,* with members of the BBC Symphony Orchestra, with arrangements written and directed by the late Johnny Douglas of RCA's *Living Strings.*

Mel enjoys making people feel good, especially through his indefatigable arsenal of quips and jokes. His family says that his joke-telling is so embedded in his DNA, that, when he opens the fridge and the light goes on, he does 20-minutes.

Mr. Calvert is a licensed pilot and contributed an article to the February 2012 issue of Aircraft Owners and Pilots Association (AOPA) Magazine.

He has also published several other books, including *Bertha's Battle,* the story of a courageous woman's winning battle against three rounds of cancer, and *A Funny Thing Happened to Me On the Way to My Funeral* — all available at AuthorsSymposium.com and Amazon.com.

Look for more edifying and fun books from his talented warp-speed mind and busy computer keyboard. Coming soon: *50 Famous People I Have Known Well or Been Close Enough To Throw A Shoe At,* and *Life After FaceBook.*

Mel presently resides in Indiana with his dynamic wife, three loving dogs and one haughty cat. They love to travel the states to visit their 6 children, 17 grandchildren and 20 great grandchildren.

DEATHS PER YEAR – GRAPHS

The graph images on the following pages illustrate the preventable deaths per year in 1998 and in the year 2018 due to tobacco use in relation to other preventable deaths.

As can be seen, tobacco-related deaths per year have not decreased, but have actually increased 2,500 deaths per year since the first Amazon edition of this book in 2010. Deaths now number a horrifying 480,000 a **YEAR** – **EVERY** year!

Special thanks to thinkprogress for the 2018 graph.

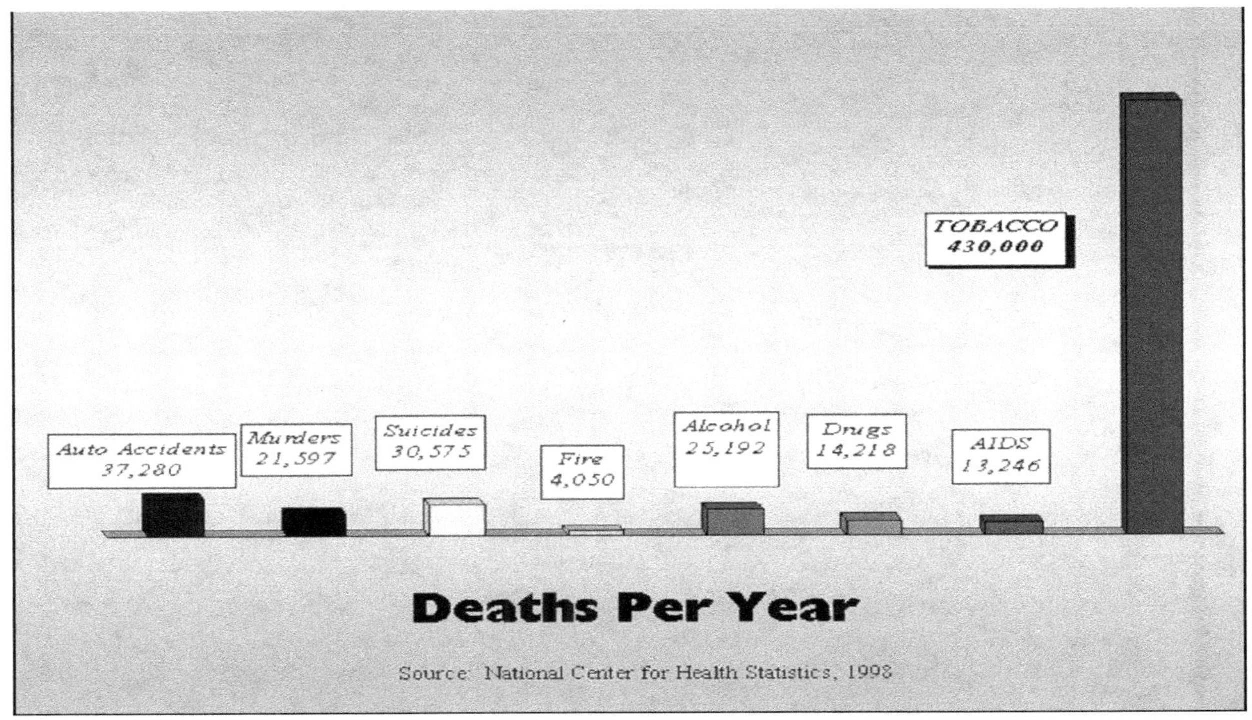

TOBACCO
430,000
Auto Accidents
37,280
Murders
21,597
Suicides
30,575
Fire
4,050
Alcohol
25,192
Drugs
14,218
AIDS
13,246
Deaths Per Year
Source: National Center for Health Statistics, 1998

SMOKING DEATHS PER YEAR, 2018

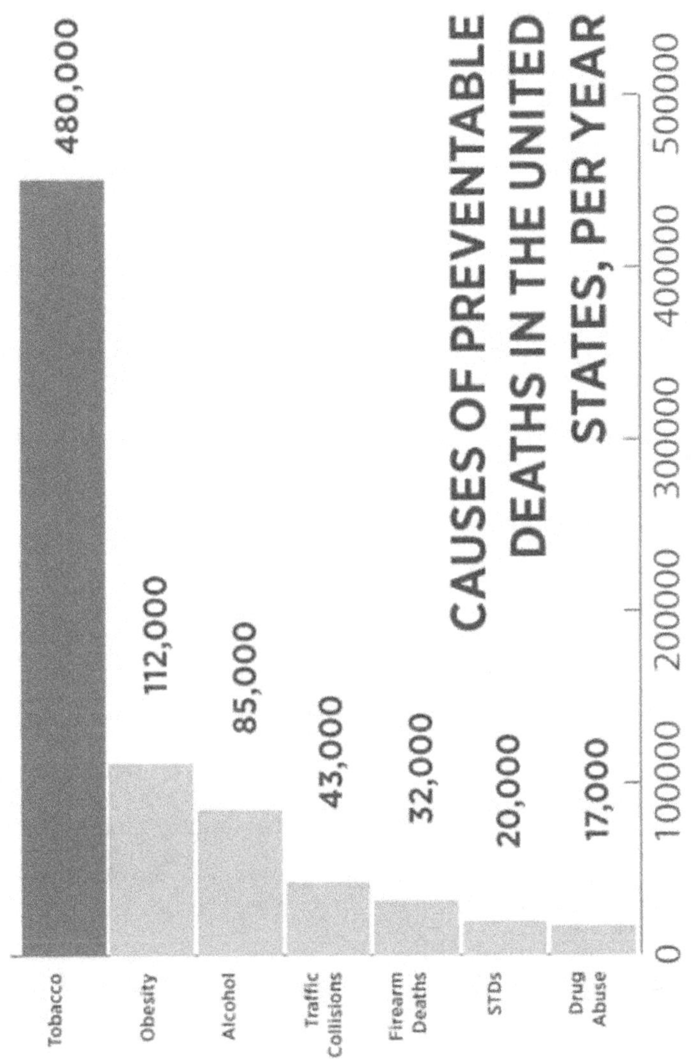

7 STEPS TO LIFE — TEAR OUT

PREPARE TO WIN!

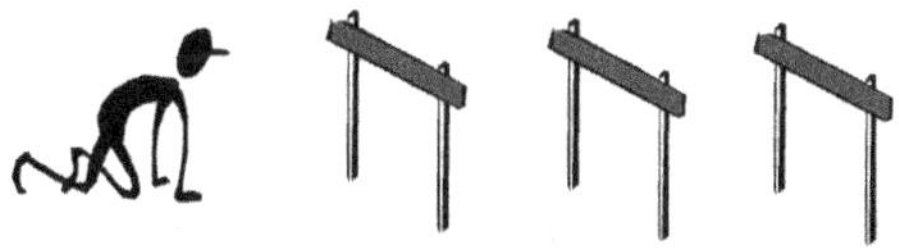

1 – ADMIT YOU'RE AN ADDICT
"MIRROR, MIRROR, ON THE WALL"

Face the mirror. Admit to yourself that you're an addict. It does no good whatsoever to admit it to anyone else until you admit it to yourself

2 – PICK YOUR Q-DAY
GO GET YOUR CALENDAR

This is another crucial part to the mental preparation. By making your **Quit Day** somewhere in the near future, that day when you say goodbye to your addiction, you can relax a little. "**I am** going to do it!" You're facing the inevitable, but not right this minute. You're giving yourself time to prepare. This is so very important.

3 – TELL THE WORLD!
GET ON 'STAGE'! USE YOUR PHONE & EMAIL

"Come on, be real." How many of us want to admit that we can't do something. Especially if we tell everyone that we're **going** to do it! The importance of this step can't be over-stressed. It will give you a lot more stamina to realize that, if you don't quit, you're not only letting yourself down, but also a lot of people who care about you and many who depend on you for their well-being.

Contact Mel Calvert · (904) 631-4898
www.AuthorsSymposium.com · Mel@AuthorsSymposium.com

4 – PICK A Q-BUDDY

KNOW WHO YOUR REAL FRIENDS ARE

Isn't it a lot more enjoyable to experience a good movie, TV show or concert *with* someone — rather than alone? Of course, it is! Therefore, a good friend or loved one who is there for you when you feel weak, your **Q-Buddy**, is equally good. If you are mates and both quitting — Hallelujah!

5 – Q-DAY EVE

START A FIRE TO PUT OUT A FIRE!

Preparing for the big day by an overindulgence in nicotine the night before may seem a bit extreme, but the logic is clear. By loading up on the drug the night before, you'll get a head start when you wake up. A cigarette is the last thing you'll want.

Also, **get rid of your remaining cigarettes** and **dispose of your ashtrays.** Your house should be smoke-free from now on. Let house visitors know that, from this day on, they go outside to smoke.

6 – Q-DAY!

KICK SOME BUTTS – KILL THE URGE!

Deep and rapid breathing at the **first** sign of craving. Remember Lamaze classes? A lot like that.

Flick your lighter. There's really no way to describe how effective this is until you do it. But do it right!

7 – NEVER SMOKE AGAIN!

AVOID YOUR PERSONAL SMOKING TRIGGERS

No coffee for several days or more, **no alcohol** for the same amount of time. **Anything that triggers your craving** should be avoided for as long as it takes to get your withdrawals under control, usually no more than a few days. This includes any situation that is conducive to a **"sociable" smoke.** Avoid them, too. If you've never tried to quit before, you'll be amazed just how quickly the cravings subside.

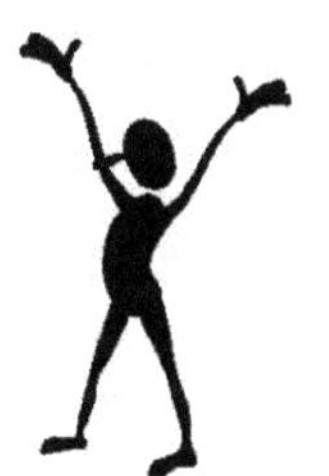